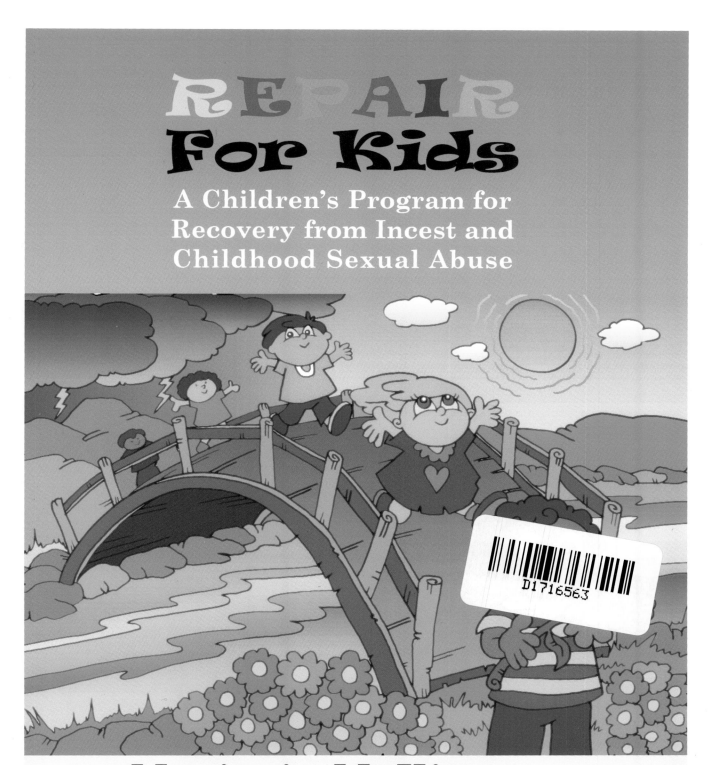

REPAIR
For Kids

A Children's Program for Recovery from Incest and Childhood Sexual Abuse

Marjorie McKinnon
Illustrated by Tom W. McKinnon

Ages 6 to 12

Book #2 in the *Growing with Love* Series

Repair For Kids: A Children's Program for Recovery from Incest and Childhood Sexual Abuse.
Book #2 in the *Growing with Love* Series.
Copyright © 2008 by Marjorie McKinnon and Tom McKinnon. All Rights Reserved.
Cover art by Kevin Scott Collier (www.KevinScottCollier.com)

Learn more about the author at www.TheLampLighters.org

First Edition: September 2008

Library of Congress Cataloging-in-Publication Data

McKinnon, Margie, 1942-
  Repair for kids : a children's program for recovery from incest and childhood sexual abuse / written by Marjorie McKinnon ; illustrated by Tom W. McKinnon.
      p. cm.
  Includes bibliographical references.
  ISBN-13: 978-1-932690-57-6 (trade paper : alk. paper)
  ISBN-10: 1-932690-57-3 (trade paper : alk. paper)
  1. Sexually abused children--Rehabilitation--Juvenile literature. 2. Incest victims--Rehabilitation--Juvenile literature. I. McKinnon, Tom W. II. Title.
  RJ507.S49M38 2008
  618.92'858360651--dc22
                          2008011510

Editing assistance from: "Righting the Writing" Editing (rightingthewriting@shaw.ca)
Special Thanks to: Catharsis Foundation -- "It's Time To Tell!"(www.catharsisfoundation.org)

Distributed by:
Baker & Taylor, Ingram Book Group, New Leaf Distributing

Published by:
Loving Healing Press
5145 Pontiac Trail
Ann Arbor, MI 48105
USA

www.LovingHealing.com or
info@LovingHealing.com
Phone 888 761 6268
Fax +1 734 663 6861

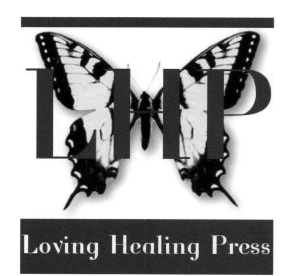

To my beloved grandchildren ......

And grandchildren everywhere

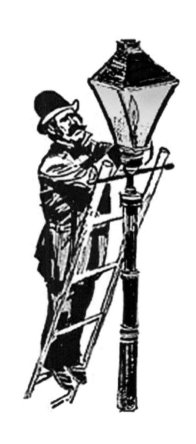

Table of Contents

Instructions for Adults

(The correct people to help children work this program are non-abusive, caring parents, relatives or therapists – but that person must be someone with whom the child feels safe.)

1. Familiarize yourself with the contents of this book and be attentive to the child's needs. Children should be encouraged to work through this book at a comfortable pace. Do not try to force their attention or cooperation; it's better to try again later.

2. Explain to the child that this program is a tool to help repair the damage done by someone who has touched them inappropriately or hurt them physically, mentally, or emotionally through sexual abuse and help them to feel happier. If there is a word they do not understand explain it to them on their level of language.

3. It is important that children get used to calling their body parts what they are: penis, vagina, breast, genital and anal area and so on. After all, we call our arm an arm and our hand a hand. Tell them that.

4. Begin reading the book to the child at a time when they are not Hungry, Angry, Lonely or Tired. It is important that you choose a time of day when they are feeling their best.

5. Pages three and four explain what Repair means. Help them to understand the general idea of each stage. As you reach each step, it will be explained further.

6. Read each page to the child, stopping to ask if they have any questions.

7. Set aside a part of each day to do the exercises with the child. Again, do them at the child's own comfortable pace. If the child is too young to write, encourage a dialogue with them regarding the exercise. The important thing is that they have an opportunity to talk about what is inside of them. They must find their voice.

8. One key to getting Repaired is repetition. Each time the child does an exercise, have him read it over. They are making their way across the bridge, which is a visual tool. Help them to keep using it as a visual tool.

9. Be patient. Be kind and caring. Be affectionate. Help the child to feel safe. It might help if they have their favorite doll, blanket, or stuffed animal with them while they are doing their exercises. Encourage them to look forward to this time. Explain that getting REPAIRED is a process, not a promise; that this book is giving them tools to help them to protect themselves as they grow older. Explain that by working the program diligently, they may have a scar but they won't continue to hurt or have "owies"; they will have been REPAIRED.

10. Keep in mind that the majority of children who are sexually assaulted are assaulted more than once. Working this program will not only help the child to heal – it will lessen their chances of being assaulted again.

11. Each child is unique and reacts differently to different forms of abuse. There are never guarantees but every effort to help the child to reclaim his/her life should be explored and tried. You should use your own judgment and take the temperament and needs of the child into consideration when teaching this program.

12. Get a copy of *He Told Me Not To Tell*, A parents' guide to talking to children about sexual assault (see Suggested Book List on p. 78) for ordering info.

RECOGNITION

ENTRY

PROCESS

AWARENESS

INSIGHT

RHYTHM

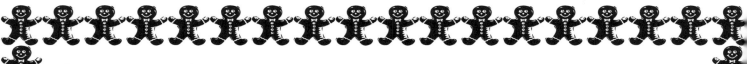

R E P A I R

Means…

R ecognition   Telling the truth about what has happened

E ntry   Making a commitment to work on the program regularly

P rocess   Learning tools and exercises to make us feel better

A wareness   Finding the puzzle pieces

I nsight   Putting the picture together so we can see that it was **not** our fault in *any* way

R hythm   Becoming our own person, special and whole

Do we want to be REPAIRed????

The Dictionary says......

"Repair means to put back into good condition after damage – to restore to a sound or healthy state by replacing a part, mending, or putting together what has been damaged."

Isn't that what we want to do?

A part of us has been broken. We want to fix it!

If something in your house breaks, it has to be repaired – doesn't it?

Our house (*meaning us*) has been broken

and we want it fixed!

Yes! We want to be REPAIRed!!!!!

Path Of The Hurting Child

At birth we were given a promise to be loved and protected.

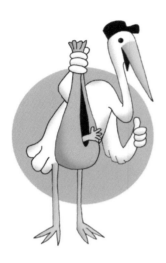
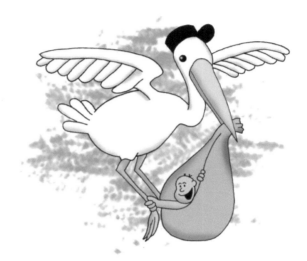

Then came the…

Bad stuff… and lions and tigers and bears and monsters ……

and Bad People ……

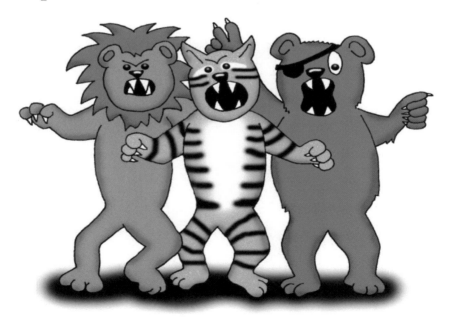

We were sad and fearful.
We didn't know which direction to turn.

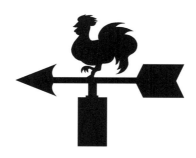

Which way? Which way? ………

Like in the Wizard of Oz where Dorothy, the Tin Man, the Scarecrow and the Lion had to find their way to the Wizard, there has to be a better path for a hurting child. We need to find our own Yellow Brick Road.

Maybe this book can help us……

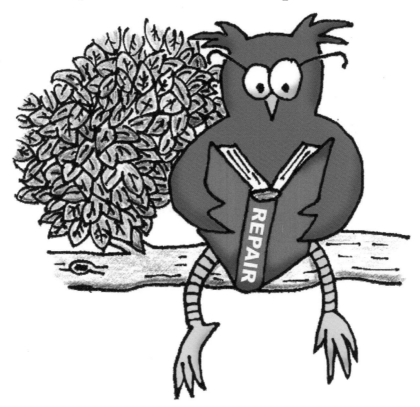

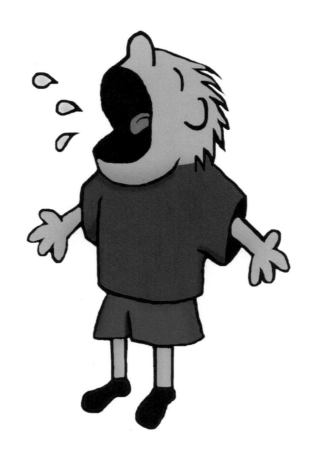

Are you a hurting child?

A hurting child is sad.

Bad things have happened to them and they don't understand why. Did they do something to cause it? They feel that they must have done something wrong, but what was it? They don't remember doing anything bad.

What can they do to feel better? What can they do to make the bad things stop and the hurt go away?

You are invited to join us
on a magical journey across

The Bridge of Recovery

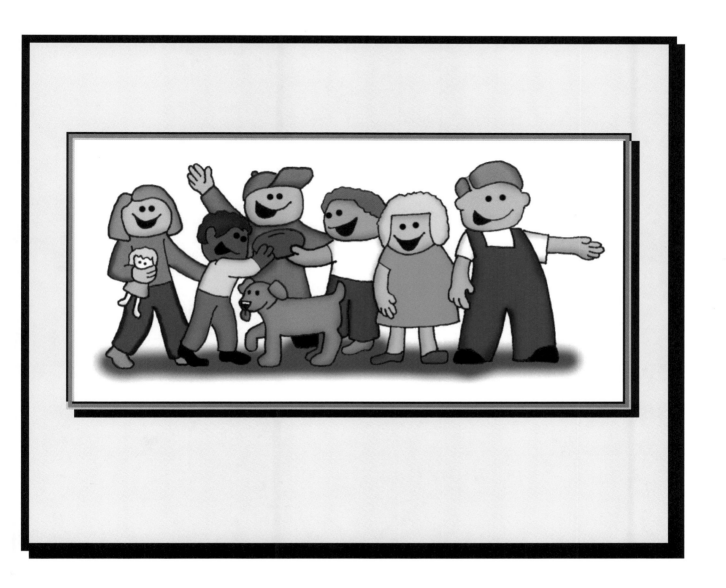

Here is a map
to help you get to
the other side
of the bridge.

It is called a

R E P A I R map.

It is a

MAGIC map!

REPAIR Map

To help you cross The Bridge of Recovery

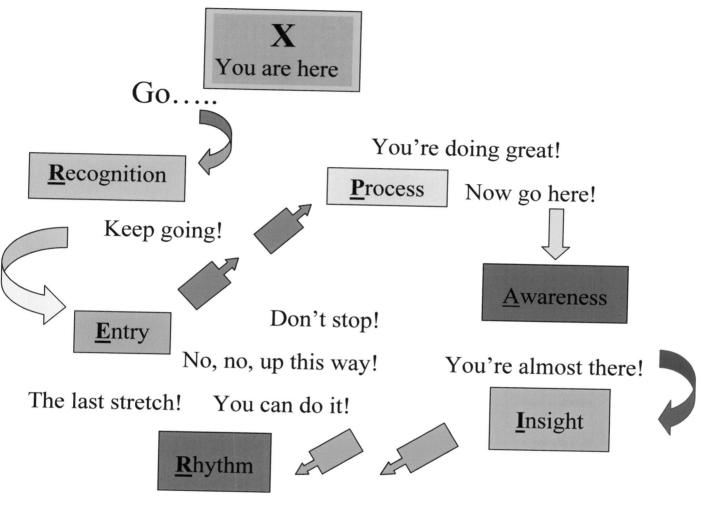

X
You are here

Go.....

Recognition

You're doing great!

Process

Now go here!

Keep going!

Awareness

Don't stop!

Entry

No, no, up this way!

You're almost there!

The last stretch!   You can do it!

Insight

Rhythm

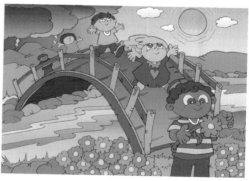

...ce you work the program and have come this far you will ...ve made it across the bridge. This program wants to make you ...onger, wiser and happier.

At the end of your journey, you will have new tools to help you to
REPAIR yourself!

How do you get there from *here?*

?????????? ??????????

By crossing...
The Bridge of Recovery

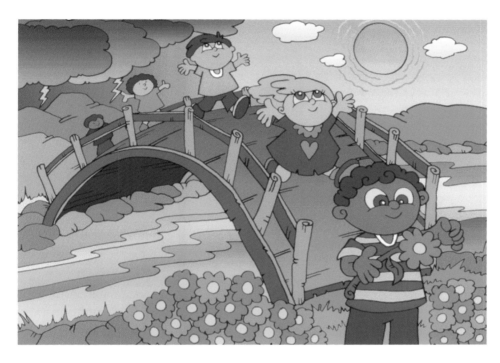

The Bridge of Recovery

It is a magical bridge. It will help you to tell your story, to talk about the bad things people did to you that hurt. You won't have to keep secrets anymore. Going across the bridge will help take you from sadness to joy, from fear to safety, from loneliness to love, from confusion to understanding. It will help take you from being a hurting child to being a happy child!

Do you want to cross the magical Bridge of Recovery?

Remember! **We have a map!**

By crossing the bridge,

you will be REPAIRed.

Remember, *'repair'* means to fix what is torn, broken, or damaged and return it to a sound or healthy state.

That's us!

We want to be fixed so that we are…..

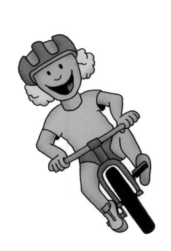

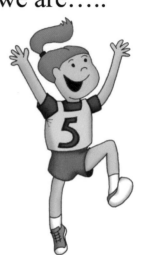

Happy, not sad

Filled with joy…………playful

Free to be ourselves

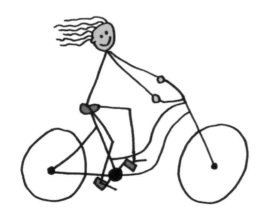

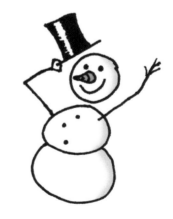

Now, it's time to start crossing the magical **Bridge of Recovery**.

Are you ready?

Take one step at a time

and

Remember what's at the other end

You are not alone

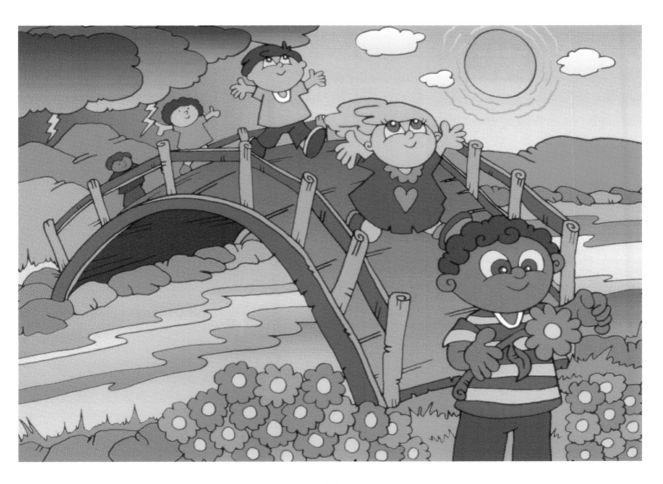

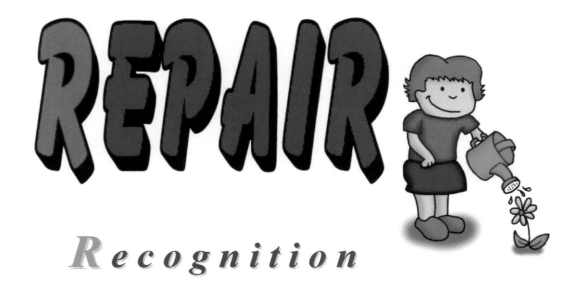

REPAIR

Recognition

Let's start with the R:

It stands for <u>R</u>ecognition. It means telling the truth and talking about anything someone did to hurt your body or try to make you feel you are a bad person when in fact you are *wonderful*.

Can you find a safe person to tell the truth to? Do **not** be afraid because it was **not** your fault. It was the fault of the person who hurt you.

Sometimes it's easier if we concentrate on what we are feeling. A happy person has not had anything bad happen to them. A sad person (one who is sad most of the time, not just once in awhile when they don't get their way) **has** had something bad done to them.

If you had a plant growing in your garden and someone stomped on it, it would not look like a healthy plant anymore. It would be flattened and trampled. But it could be made healthy and happy again if you watered it, talked to it and cared for it – it can be REPAIRED.

You are like that plant. Someone has trampled on you and now you need to be nurtured. But first you must talk about anything bad that was done to you. Recognition is the first step. Telling the truth will make you feel stronger, more powerful. It doesn't matter if someone told you not to tell. They were wrong and now you are going to talk about it.

First, let's do an exercise called, *What am I Feeling?*

What am I feeling?

Feelings just **are**. They are not right or wrong, good or bad. It is what we **do** with our feelings that we need to look at.

*What are **you** feeling?*

Write down as many feelings as you can think of. If you need to, write some down for each day of the week. For example: Monday I was angry, Tuesday I was mostly happy except when I had a fight with my sister, and so on.

_____

_____

_____

_____

_____

_____

_____

_____

_____

Checklist
to find out if we are a hurting child

I have trouble sleeping. _____

I get angry a lot. _____

I feel shameful. _____

I need to please people in order to feel good about myself. _____

I am fearful of certain people. _____

I have trouble saying **<u>No</u>**. _____

I want someone to protect me. _____

I have nightmares a lot, usually the same ones over and over. _____

I am sick a lot. _____

I am needy a lot. _____

I cry a lot, but I don't know why. _____

Check the ones that apply to you the <u>most</u>

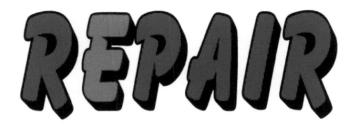

REPAIR

Next is the **E** *...which stands for*

Entry

It means we are going to make a promise to ourselves to read this book every day.

It means we will do the exercises on a daily basis.

It means we will not keep secrets when something bad happens to us. When someone asks us to do something (even if it's a family member) and we get that "yucky" feeling, we will tell someone we trust.

It means we are going to bond with healthy behavior.

It means we are going to learn to set healthy boundaries.

It means we will learn to say **NO** when it needs to be said.

It means we are going to learn the C word, Commitment

" *Commitment* "

means a pledge or promise.

Now, raise your right hand
and repeat after me…

"I give my word that I will stay on this bridge and keep working my way to the other side where I can be happy."

Now that was easy, wasn't it?

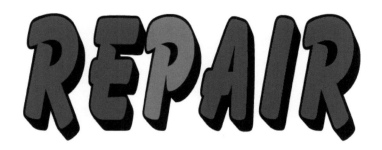

The **P** in Repair stands for......

Process

Process means......

Gradual changes that lead towards......

Getting to the other side of the bridge!!!

To being REPAIRed!!

In order to get there, picture our bridge and what lies on the other side of it.

It's time to put on big people pants and begin our incredible journey across the bridge. We have a magic map and fun exercises to help us!

Let's start with a question…………

What is on this side of the bridge, where you are now???

Sadness

Tears

Loneliness

Fear

No one will like me

Feeling ugly

Feeling stupid

Feeling I've done something wrong

Fear of abandonment

Feeling ashamed

Do you want these things in your life?

No! No! No! No! No!

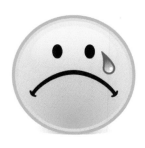

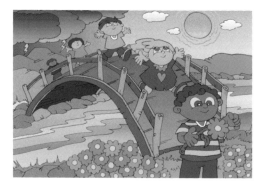

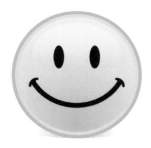

Here is where
you are now

Here is where
you want to be

This is what waits for you
on the other side of the bridge…

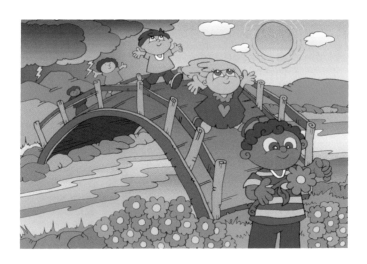

Happiness

No more fear

Acceptance

Feeling good about myself

No more feeling ugly

Knowing I deserve kindness

Knowing I haven't done anything wrong

Everyone likes me

I'm smart, smart, smart

No more bad secrets

Do you want these things in your life?

Yes! Yes! Yes! Yes! Yes!!!!!!!!!!!!!!!

Let's start our journey with a
Magic Mirror

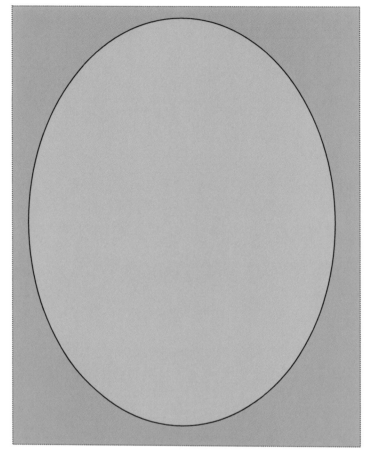

My Magic Mirror

Mirror, Mirror on the wall,
Who's the fairest of them all?

ME!

Before working on our Magic Mirror, we have one more thing to do…

Healthy and Unhealthy Messages

Some people say ugly things just to hurt people. It is not right and it would be wonderful if no one did this, but some people are just not nice. If someone always says mean and ugly things to us, it makes us feel shame – even if we know what they're saying is not true! When people do this they are actually saying that *they* are not nice – not us.

It is best to stay away from these people!

We are going to help you get rid of these ugly messages that ugly people say and replace them with wonderful, healthy replacement words.

In the following exercise, write the unhealthy message that someone said and then write a TRUE healthy replacement message about yourself.

For example:

Unhealthy Message	**Healthy Replacement Message**
You're so stupid, you never do anything right.	*I am very smart and I do many things right.*
_____	_____
_____	_____
_____	_____
_____	_____
_____	_____
_____	_____
_____	_____
_____	_____

Now, let's begin working with your …
Magic Mirror

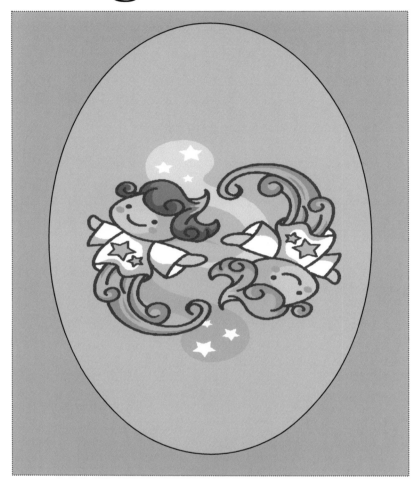

My Magic Mirror

Tape a picture of yourself in the center

of your real mirror at home.

This is now *your* Magic Mirror.

Tape happy, positive messages

around the picture of you …

For example:

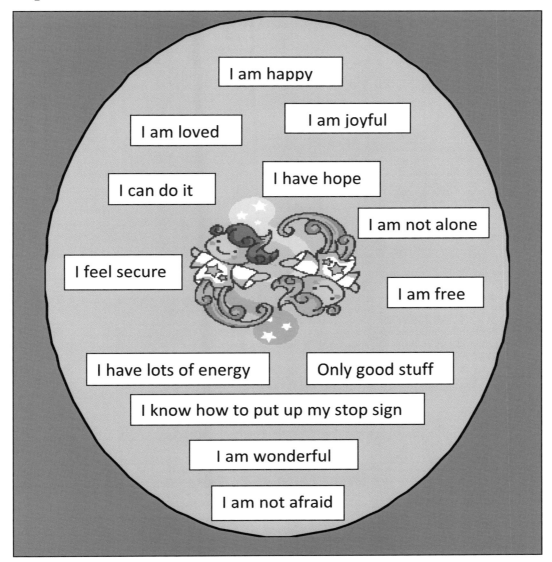

Doing the Magic Mirror exercise is fun!
We need fun! It helps us to feel better.

Read your happy words out loud every time you look into the mirror.

Starting on the next page, I have given you suggestions of positive messages to feel about yourself, but if you find some on your own or think of any, write them down and tape them to your mirror as well. To be effective, you must say them every day, all of them...
And <u>know</u> they are true!!!

Remember your promise!

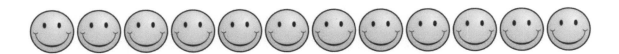

Suggestions for my Magic Mirror

I am a wonderful person.

When other people hurt me, it's because they are bad, not me.

I can be whatever I want when I grow up.

I am stronger than I think I am.

I am smart.

I know how to say "NO!" to bad things.

I know how to ask for help when I need help.

I deserve respect as much as anyone else does.

Many people love me because I'm so lovable.

I am a winner.

I am considerate and kind.

I am never alone because God is always with me.

My Guardian Angel watches out for me.

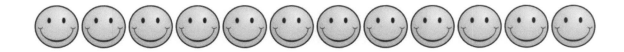

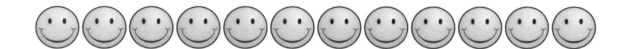

I am special.

It's OK to cry when I feel sad.

It's OK to have all my different feelings.

It's OK to talk about my feelings.

Sometimes I'm afraid, but it's OK

I will smile, because my world is going to be all right.

When I make a mistake, I can forgive myself.

When I get angry, it's OK to talk about it.

It's OK to feel angry, but not okay to hurt others.

I can say I'm sorry and still feel OK about me.

I need love and I'm not afraid to say that.

When I grow up, I can be everything I want to be.

I will learn to move through my pain and heal.

I have people who care about me in my life.

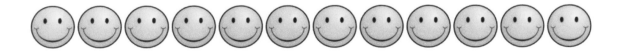

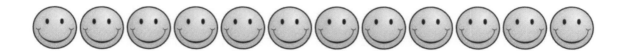

Sometimes bad things happen, but I can heal from them.

The only thing that's the end of the world is … the end of the world.

If something bad happens to me, I can talk about it to healthy people.

Talking about the bad things makes me feel better.

_____

_____

_____

_____

_____

_____

_____

Ask someone who knows you VERY WELL for more ideas!

Dear Diary...

Write a private letter to your Inner Child

Big People call this a Journal or a Diary – we will write to our Inner Child in our Diary. We all have an Inner Child; that secret, private part of ourselves that knows everything, that loves us completely and unconditionally, and is there when we need them.

Write a letter to your Inner Child about everything that is in your heart – whether you are sad and why, or happy and why, what is troubling you, and so on. Keep these letters in a secret place where no one can find them because they are ONLY between you and your Inner Child.

Putting your thoughts and troubles on paper can help ease a lot of pain. For example, if your teacher hollered at you for something you didn't do and it made you feel bad, you might write...

> *"Dear Me (or Dear Diary), I am very angry at my teacher for hollering at me. I hate being yelled at, especially when I didn't do anything wrong. It is so unfair! But I know now that it is really a statement about my teacher (having a bad day, being a bully, are just plain grumpy and taking it out on someone smaller than them – or whatever...) It was never about me."*

By the time you've finished writing the letter, you'll feel much better. Sometimes our Inner Child can help us to work out a problem when we write our letters to them.

I'm feeling better and better with every day that passes. I'll never be alone again because now I have my Inner Child to write to as often as I want to.

Draw pictures of what you are feeling...

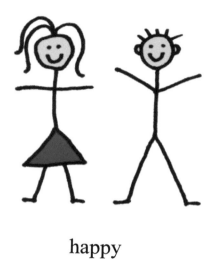

happy

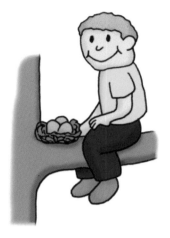

excited

or maybe…

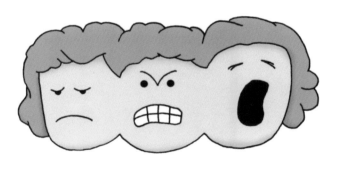

sad   angry   very unhappy

or worse….

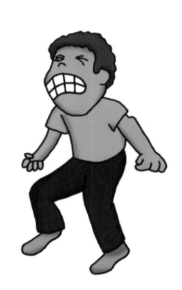

VERY ANGRY!

Draw pictures of your life.
Be sure to include any pictures of anyone touching your private parts.
If you are right-handed, draw these pictures with your left hand.
If you are left-handed, draw these pictures with your right hand.
Don't worry if you can't draw very well. Most people can't.
Stick figures will do just fine.

Draw pictures here...

Draw pictures here too…

Use separate paper for more room to draw as many pictures as you want.

- 35 -

We also need to talk about…

Shame

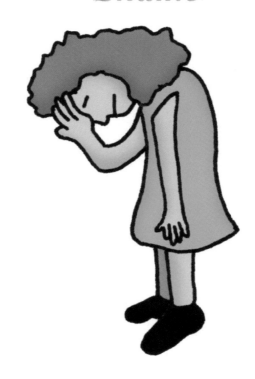

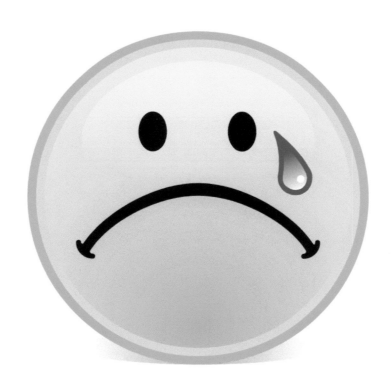

Hurting children feel shame, that hot rush to our body that makes us feel bad. Shame is embarrassing and we really want to hide it. We feel like we've done something bad or wrong. Shame hurts but with time and help, we can stop feeling shame and not hurt so much. We may be children in pain but we can take care of our own hurt – we can do something to help ourselves to feel better because we are smart.

That is what this Repair program is all about!

It's like going to the doctor to get well,

except we can be our own doctor.

Because we are smart!

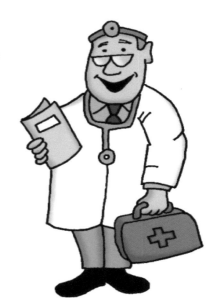

Then...

One day, we will no longer wear a sad face…

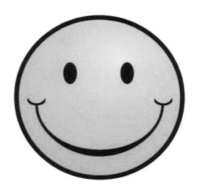

We will wear a Happy Face!!!

Shame is *usually* caused by guilt. Guilt is our conscience telling us we did something wrong. Sometimes this guilt is deserved but sometimes…

IT IS NOT DESERVED!

An example of deserved guilt is if we forget to feed our dog and Mom gives us a lecture – we may feel shame and believe that Mom sees us as a lesser person.

Do we deserve that?

If we did forget to feed the dog and that is our job, we probably deserved the lecture – and the guilt and shame.

Everyone has accidentally done something they were sorry for. In this example, shame helps to remind us to do better next time. It is part of the learning experience of life!

From the time we are born...

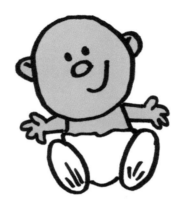

Our bodies are our own!

They belong to us!

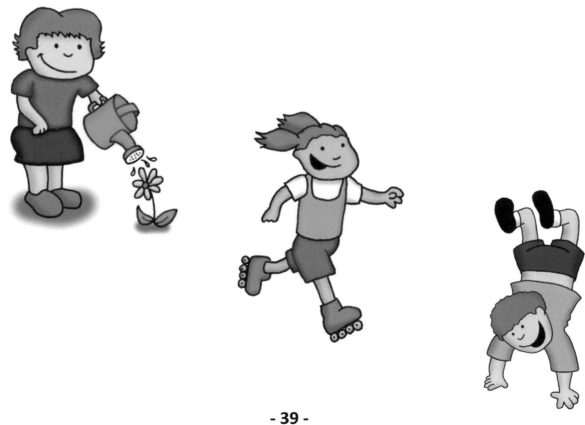

If someone touches our private parts in a *shameful* manner when we don't want them to, the shame that we feel crawls over us like a giant monster. Our private parts are in that part of our body that we keep covered when we go swimming. These are called private parts because they belong to us alone.

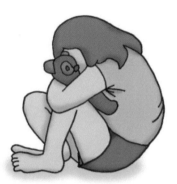

We think it must be *our* fault if someone touches our private parts, but it is **NOT**! No one has the right to touch any part of your body that you don't want them to – *ever*! When they do, the shame is so great that we cannot tell anyone, mostly because we think we were bad or it was our fault.

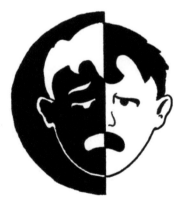

Sometimes the person who touched our private parts is someone in our family. This makes the shame even greater. **NO ONE** has the right to hurt you. You have the right to say **"NO!"** and to phone someone you trust for protection. If you don't know anyone, you can call the police on the telephone and they will help you.

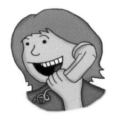

You are **NOT** the bad person; the person who hurt you was bad. They are bad people and must learn not to hurt you, *or anyone else*, again. You must be strong and protect your own body. This book will help you to be strong and REPAIR the damage that bad people did to you.

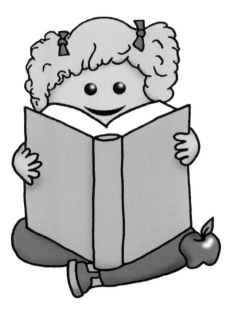

You are a wonderful child of love and you are a gift to the world! This book helps you to see your own wonderfulness. Lots of people are waiting to protect you if you let them – but they can't read your mind – you just have to let them know that you need help.

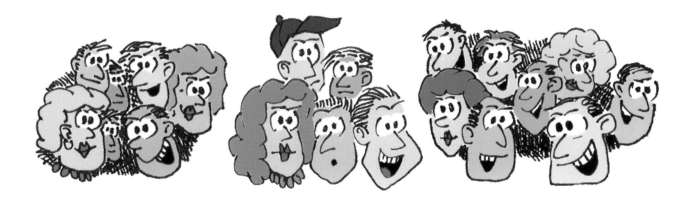

Qualities other people think I have

Some times, people act less than perfect! Other qualities are just part of being human. But sometimes big people want us to think we have a lot of imperfect qualities. We will find out later that this is just **not true.**

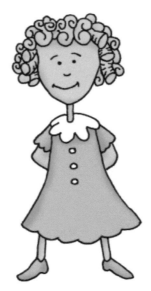

(Psst! This is you!)

Some days we just get out of bed on the wrong side...☺

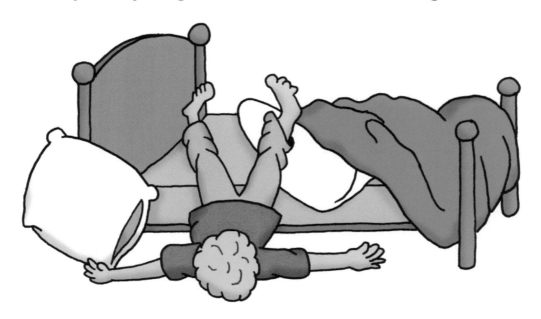

Ooops!

Maybe we forgot to make our bed. That's not a big deal. You've probably seen mom forget to make her bed a lot. But she thinks it means you did something bad. In fact, she may be feeling guilty about not making the bed herself and decided to take it out on you. These qualities do not belong to you. They are a reflection of what I call "big people problems". Let's make a list of possibilities!

When I was little, if my mom put something on my plate I didn't like, I fed it to our dog that was lying under the table. My mom didn't think that was funny. When my son was four years old, he hid under the bed so that when I went to make it he grabbed both my ankles. I let out a scream and he crawled out from under the bed and said, "Am in trouble?" Then I laughed so hard that he figured out he wasn't in trouble.

But sometimes big people have so many worries or problems that they lose their sense of humor and they complain about things we do that they don't like. Let's make a list of these

Qualities other people *think I have* that need to be changed...

_____

_____

_____

_____

_____

See! It's a short list.

Save this little list for now because we have a very important job to do with it later.

Take a Break

You should take a break from your determined work towards self-repair whenever you begin to feel tired or overwhelmed. Be good to yourself, and above all else, love yourself. If you need to take time out from doing the exercises in this book, allow yourself to take a break and to breathe...

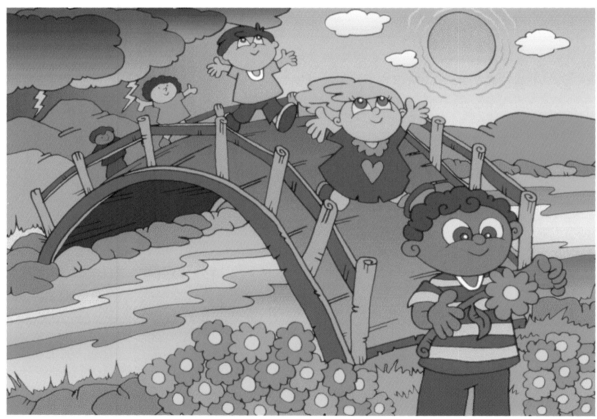

(Bridge of Recovery - Remember??)

As you travel across your Bridge of Recovery, some tips and reminders might help you in case you're having trouble...

Tips to help you

make your

journey…

Take care of yourself!
Whenever you are feeling.....

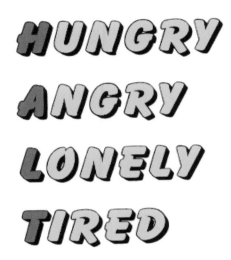

.....and you will soon feel better!

Think of 4 examples of ways to help overcome each

For example:
   Hungry – eat a peanut butter and jelly sandwich
   Angry – punch my pillow ten times
   Lonely – hug my pet
   Tired – take a nap

HUNGRY	ANGRY	LONELY	TIRED
_____	_____	_____	_____
_____	_____	_____	_____
_____	_____	_____	_____
_____	_____	_____	_____

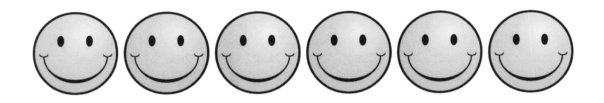

The Attitude of Gratitude

Sometimes when we only remember bad things, we can forget about all the things that make us feel happy. Make a list of everything you are grateful for – no matter how small.

For example: I have a terrific bedroom. My grandma and I are real close and I am very grateful for her. The sun was shining today, and so on.

_____

_____

_____

_____

_____

_____

_____

You might need *lots more* paper for this list!! ☺

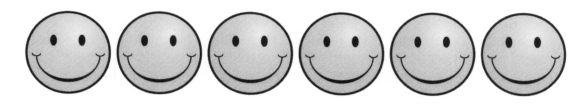

Courage Songs

As you journey across the Bridge of Recovery, you may feel afraid, or sad, or angry, or lonely at times. But sometimes, music has its own special magic that can make us feel better.

Do you have favorite songs that you like to sing? Songs that make you feel good when you sing them?

List some of your favorite songs here and sing them often. They will help you cross that bridge.

_____   _____

_____   _____

_____   _____

_____   _____

_____   _____

_____   _____

_____   _____

_____   _____

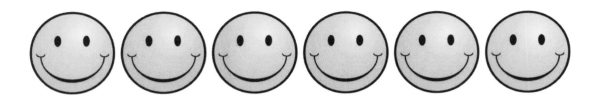

Pamper Yourself

What makes you feel good inside? A bubble bath? Eating popcorn and watching a Disney movie? Reading? Helping mom bake a cake? Playing games? Make a list of things that make you feel good and whenever you start to feel sad, pick one of them and do it. You will start feeling happier right away.

_____

_____

_____

_____

_____

_____

_____

Remind yourself

Look into your Magic Mirror…
And read it over and over and over and over and …
Remember?

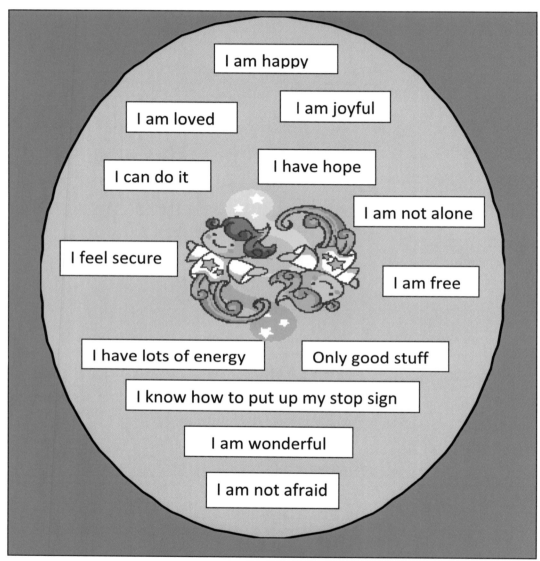

I am happy

I am joyful

I am loved

I can do it

I have hope

I am not alone

I feel secure

I am free

I have lots of energy

Only good stuff

I know how to put up my stop sign

I am wonderful

I am not afraid

Happy words on a Magic Mirror

Write a letter to your Inner Child, that small *you* that is waiting for the two of you to meet. Also, make a wish list to help you to *know* what will make you happy—many people are unhappy because they don't know that. They don't have a clue what will make them feel better.

Saying NO!

This part is fun!

Let's start with….

Practicing when to say **NO!**

Saying **NO** when it is the right thing to do is a way to make us feel more powerful – and strong enough to keep walking across that bridge.

It is another way to set our own personal boundary

Saying NO when Mom asks us to clean our room is not the right time. We are responsible for cleaning our own room just like mom is responsible for cleaning hers.

Saying NO when a friend asks us to steal candy at the store is a right time…

Saying NO if someone touches us in a private place is not only a right time to say NO,

it is extremely important to say NO.

Make a list of times when it is okay to say NO and when it is not okay to say NO. Maybe mom or a friend can help you with this list.

It is okay to say NO when....

_____

_____

_____

_____

_____

_____

It is __not__ okay to say NO when....

_____

_____

_____

_____

_____

Boundaries

A <u>boundary</u> is a limit you set to protect yourself.

If someone asks you to do something but you're not sure if you want to, you have the right to say, "I'll think about it and let you know."

If someone asks you a question that is personal or private – and *none of their business* – you have the right to say, "Why do you ask?" or "That's kind of a personal question." Don't let anyone bully or manipulate you.

Bullying is when someone is mean or cruel to someone who is weaker. For example, someone who calls you a cruel name is trying to bully you.

Manipulate means to control – *in an unfair way* – by someone who is trying to get their own way. For example, if someone you thought was a good friend says, "I don't like that kid and if you were really my friend you wouldn't like that kid either!" Your answer might be, "It's too bad you don't like that kid but I think that kid is a really neat person."

Stand in front of a mirror and practice giving answers you could give to someone who tries to bully or manipulate you. You might want to say, "I'm sorry you feel that way but I know it's not true." Then you can turn your back and walk away. The more you practice this in front of a mirror, the more powerful you'll get. Learning this kind of power is like giving yourself a gift.

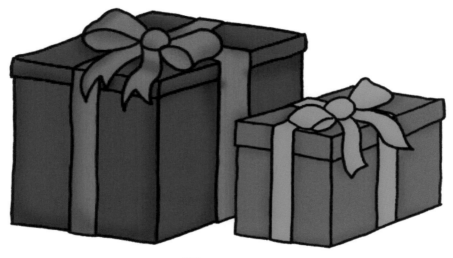

Think of other ways to set your own boundaries. If someone is working through this program with you, practice with each other. Make believe you are setting your boundary – then switch roles. A good friend, especially someone you can trust and who understands what you are going through, is really awesome to have!

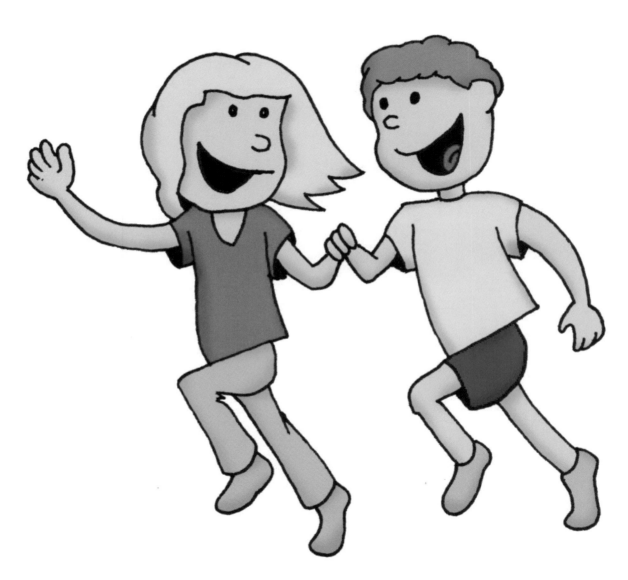

Good Friends

Ways to set <u>YOUR</u> boundaries

WHEN	HOW
_____	_____
_____	_____
_____	_____
_____	_____
_____	_____
_____	_____
_____	_____
_____	_____
_____	_____
_____	_____
_____	_____
_____	_____
_____	_____
_____	_____
_____	_____
_____	_____

Don't you feel more powerful already?

Be sure to read this list every day.

Add new ways whenever you think of them.

Now it's time to meet your...
Inner Child

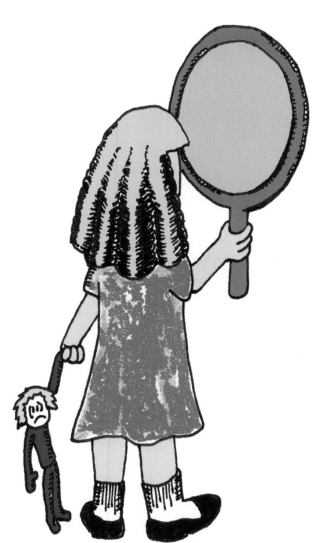

There is a child inside each of us,

who knows the truth of what happened,

that child is waiting

inside you,

with a sad face

for you to set free

so they can tell their story

and put a Band-Aid on their pain

to make the pain go away

and begin to heal

and be a happy child again!

Your Inner Child

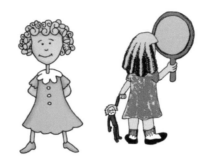

Your Inner Child has been waiting to be set free – by you. Find a favorite, quiet place – like maybe under a tree in your back yard, or in your room – and sit quietly. Breathe deeply. Close your eyes and picture that child inside of you. That Inner Child and is waiting for you in a place of sadness, a place of darkness, a place with no protection.

Picture your Inner Child after you've been working through part of Repair. Imagine this child smiling. Picture the two of you as if two close friends are finally meeting to help set each other free.

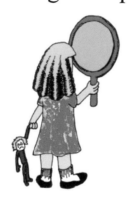

Do you see who is *really* looking into the magic mirror?

This is your Inner Child!

Can you picture yourself giving your Inner Child *a big hug*?

Now we are ready for the next step in ...

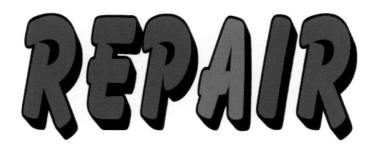

Awareness

Awareness means knowing, being watchful, sensible. It is that part of us that is able to be AWARE of what is going on around us and in the world. **Awareness** is another magical sense we all have – but not everyone uses.

> *For example: If we smell chocolate baking in the kitchen, our awareness tells us that mom is probably baking a cake.*

There are lots of things that we should be aware of. As we work our way across the magical Bridge of Recovery, we will become more aware and wiser. It will be like opening doors and finding 'truth'.

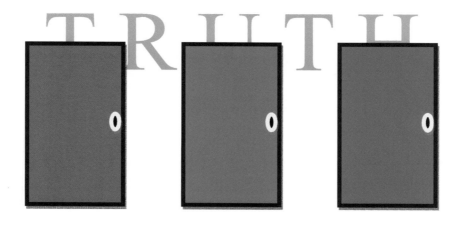

"Awareness" means...

✓ **Being smart and using your head**

✓ **Thinking things through**

✓ **Knowing what's going on around you**

✓ **Using your mind to see ahead and into the future**

✓ **Knowing what you're feeling**

What are some of the ways **you** use your magic Awareness senses?

> *For example: "using your mind to see ahead and into the future" might be, "If I take a cookie after mom told me not to, she will probably make me do a timeout or something else to punish me, so I better not take any."*

_____

_____

_____

_____

_____

_____

_____

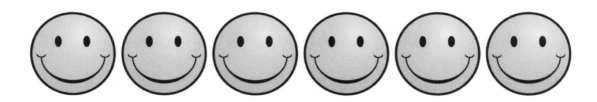

Family Systems

When we are children we don't have much choice about the family we belong to – and not all families are happy families.

☹ **Sometimes, Dad is bossy and no one gets to say a thing about anything.**

☹ **Sometimes, mom is sad because she doesn't know how to set boundaries.**

☹ **Sometimes, our family follows the rules of our church – right or wrong – because we're supposed to even if sometimes the rules might not seem right to us.**

☹ **Sometimes, someone in our family drinks too much alcohol and they walk and talk different – sometimes it makes them mean.**

☹ **Sometimes, we hear about other people in our family who have been touched in a yucky manner in their private parts or maybe have done it to other children.**

These are just a few of the "sometimes" that could make up our family system – and sometimes our family systems hurt us but it is not our fault – it is the fault of the family system.

Being aware of the truth makes us stronger and gives us the freedom to be ourselves. Accepting the truth helps us to realize that if someone hurts us, it is their doing and their fault – it is NEVER our fault.

We now know that if anyone touches our private places, we can scream our heads off or call the police. We now KNOW that we have the right to say NO when someone tries to hurt us and we KNOW that we have the right to ask for help from anyone we can trust.

This coming to Awareness is an awesomely wonderful thing. It means we are beginning to put together the pieces of the puzzle, the puzzle we started when we began this program.

The puzzle contained broken pieces of us,
    pieces we needed to gather together,
       repair, and put back together,
          to make us complete and happy again.

You should be starting to feel better already!!!!

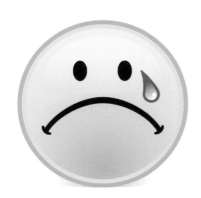
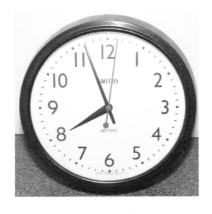
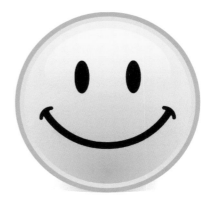

Here is where
you are now

with
time

Here is where
you want to be

Take time to breathe…

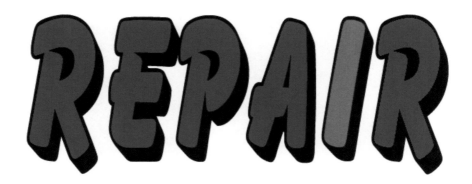

Insight

First, let's recap…

We started with **Recognition**, where we learned to know the truth and to tell the truth, to talk about anything someone has done to hurt us.

Next came **Entry**; we entered into a commitment (remember raising your hand and making a promise) to work hard to get to the other side of the magical *Bridge of Recovery*. We promised to make entries into this book and work through the exercises to help ourselves feel better.

Then we talked about **Process**, where we learned exercises and easy things to do to feel better about ourselves. We were becoming stronger!

Happy, not sad!

Then we began building our **Awareness**…
>   that special part of us that gives us super magical powers to know things like…

☺   knowing what we feel
☺   knowing we can think ahead
☺   knowing what is right and wrong.

We were becoming very smart, something that even some 90-year-old people never become!

And we did it all by ourselves!
Hooray for us!
Now let's do some really fun exercises!

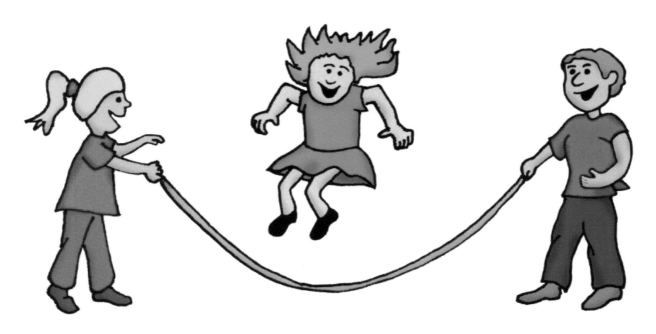

No, we're not going to play –
this will make us happier than playing.

Insight is the most magical of all the steps of REPAIR!
It's like having x-ray vision. Insight is the special power to see what makes us angry and sad.

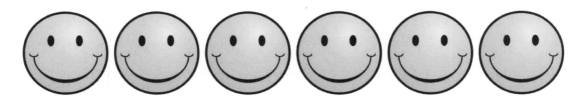

Real Love Qualities

Everyone has their own idea of what makes them feel loved. For example: hugs, laughter, playtime or reading stories – whatever makes them feel loved.

Make a list of what kind of "real love" qualities you'd like to receive. An example might be: "I feel loved when someone bakes cookies for me," or "I feel loved when I am not ignored when I ask a question." Make your list realistic. Asking for $100 a week allowance may not be considered real love and eating all the candy you want wouldn't mean real love either.

My list of "real love" qualities:
I feel loved when ...

_____

_____

_____

_____

_____

_____

_____

Don't be afraid to share this list – no one can read your mind.

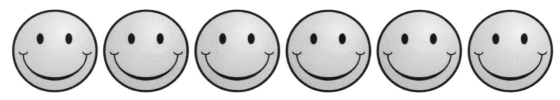

My Wonderful Qualities

Everyone has good qualities that make them who they are. But when we are hurting, we sometimes have qualities we don't like about ourselves. They are the result of being unhappy or angry or unable to tell people why we are hurting. But there are also lots of good things about our selves – we're talking about our wonderful qualities.

Examples of wonderful qualities: you are caring and loving, you are kind to animals, you do your chores when you're supposed to, you are a good friend to others, and so on.
Let's list them now.

I am:

_____

_____

_____

_____

_____

_____

_____

_____

_____

And more of my great qualities are…

_____

_____

_____

_____

_____

This list can be as short or as long as you choose to make it – but it really is an endless list if you take an honest look at yourself. See how wonderful you are! But if you can't see your own wonderfulness, talk to someone who loves you and someone you trust – ask them what some of your wonderful qualities are. Promise to read this list every day so you don't forget how wonderful you are. You will probably discover more things to add too! *That's how wonderful you are!*

Remember that list of qualities other people think you have that need to be changed? It's time to crumple up that list and throw it in the trash. It was someone else's opinions and didn't belong to you.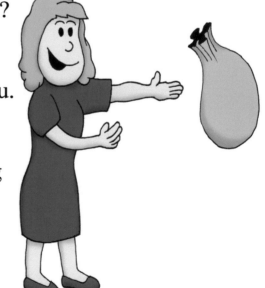

Besides, you are busy with the wise words on your Magic Mirror and living with happy thoughts about yourself.

So take that list and toss it in the trash. **You don't need it anymore!**
!

Remember when we said earlier that your body belongs to you? Here are some pictures that might remind you....

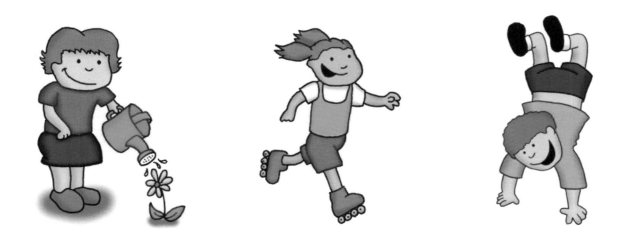

Since your body is your own, that means you get to say whether anyone touches you or how they touch you. If someone wants to give you a kiss and you don't want them to, just say, "No thank you. I'm not comfortable with that." If someone wants you to sit on their lap and you don't like that idea either, you can say, "I'm too big to sit on people's laps." See? If someone tries to cross your boundaries on anything that has to do with your body, (whether it is someone who wants to watch you bathe or someone who wants to take a nap with you, or anything that makes you feel yucky) you have the right to go to someone you trust and who makes you feel safe and tell them about it IMMEDIATELY. When you say NO – you mean it!

<u>Our bodies are our own!</u>

<u>They belong to us!</u>

Now for the BIGGIE, the last step in our journey across the magical Bridge of Recovery...

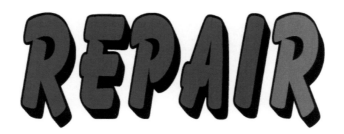

Rhythm

Rhythm is the last "R" in Repair. It is a movement marked by a natural flow – like the rhythm of nature; first is spring, then comes summer, then autumn and then winter arrives – then the rhythm is repeated. That is a natural flow, the rhythm of the seasons.

Our breathing has a natural rhythm too. We breathe in, we breathe out – in then out – in and out …. When we are asleep, the rhythm of our breathing is healthy, deep and slow. When we are afraid, the rhythm of our breathing is unhealthy, shallow and fast.

Each of us is born with rhythms and natural flows in other ways too – a natural rhythm that is imprinted in us that makes us unique. Some people go to sleep early every night, some are shy, and some people can't sit still for a minute, etc – no two humans are alike – just as no two snowflakes are alike. We are each special in our own way and our natural rhythms belong to us.

They mean, **"THIS IS ME!"**

But when someone hurts us, touches the private parts of our bodies or shames us by making us take our clothes off when we don't want to, or does anything to us that makes us have that "yucky" feeling, not only is the natural rhythm of our breathing affected but our other natural rhythms are interrupted as well.

For example, if we were once naturally happy, out-going and laughed a lot, we might suddenly stop laughing after being hurt. We might become quiet and withdrawn.

If we felt comfortable and safe in our bedrooms but then someone hurt us in our bedroom, that feeling of comfort and safety might change to dread and fear of going into our bedrooms.

But guess what! We have been moving across that Bridge of Recovery using our magic map of Repair and every day we have been getting stronger. We started moving from a place of fear to confidence, from feeling sadness to feeling happiness and joy, from shame to feeling good about ourselves. We are returning to our natural rhythms, the ones that were damaged when we were molested or hurt by someone.

Now we can do the most wonderful exercise of all. It's called,

"Who Am I?"

Here you can list all the things about yourself that describes the real and happy YOU. Leave nothing out. Read it every day and you will begin to return to your own happy self.

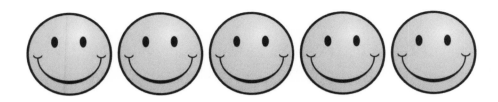

Who Am I?

Describe the **real** you. List everything you can think about yourself.

For example: Are you playful? Do you like the forest or do you like the beach? Are you funny?

_____

_____

_____

_____

_____

_____

_____

_____

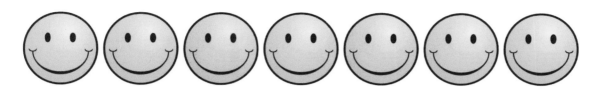

My Wish List

Now you have one last exciting exercise to do…

Write down everything you would like to be, to have and to learn in your life. (In other words, everything that will make you happy!) Remember, we started this wish list earlier…

Include everything you want to happen to you – not only as you grow up but after you are an adult. It doesn't matter if it seems silly or impossible! Wish lists help you KNOW what will make you happy – many people are unhappy because they don't know. They don't have a clue what will make them feel happy.

Add to your Wish List any time you want to. You don't have to finish it now, but the important thing is to read it and remind yourself every day of what you are wishing for, even if you only have only one thing on it.

Your list of everything you would like to be, have and learn. Include your wishes for when you are grown up as well as for now.

Leave nothing out!

You should be able to think of lots of things that will make <u>YOU</u> happy – if you can't, you need to try harder...

but never quit trying!

I wish:

_____

_____

_____

_____

_____

_____

_____

_____

_____

Guess what???

You made it!

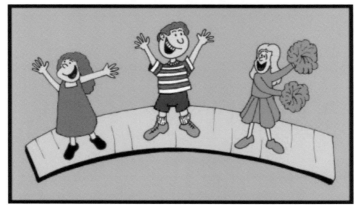

Not only have you crossed the

Bridge of Recovery...

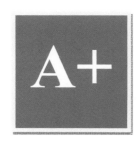

You have gotten the best grade ever!!

You now have the tools to be happy

And surround yourself with healthy people...

Nice people who make wise choices,

Like you!!

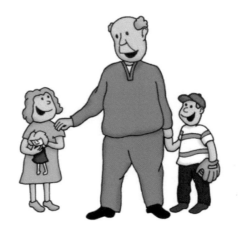

You and your Inner Child have taken all the bad things that happened to you and thrown them in the trashcan – the garbage belongs to the bad people who hurt you…

Not to you!

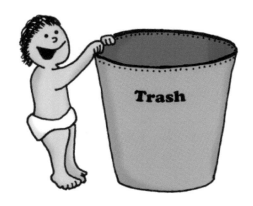

You have gone from being a ghost of your former self…

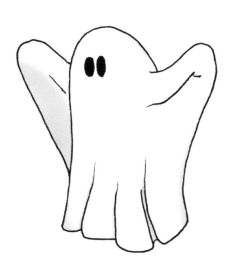

To being the **REAL** you…

Happy and not afraid.

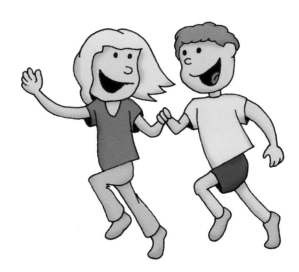

You know how to set your own boundaries.

You learned how to say **NO!**

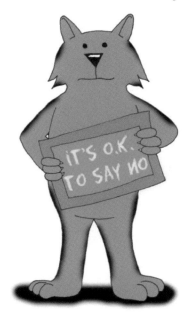

You learned how to deal with problems.

Has this **REPAIR** program helped you to be aware that you are in control of your own happiness?

Do you now realize that no one can really take your happiness away from you?

Even if they try!

Are you now aware of your super powers that protect you from the effects of bad things?

YOU DID IT!

You are now strong and powerful.

Being **REPAIRED** makes us feel terrific!

You now have tools to help make healthy choices and set boundaries.

That "owie" is now almost forgotten.

Jump for joy!!

    Wag your tail!!

Take a bow!

    HOORAY FOR YOU!

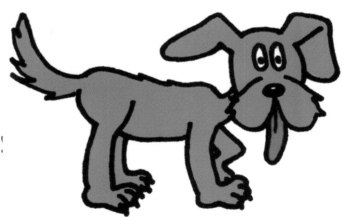

YOU ARE ABSOLUTELY WONDERFUL!!!

The Serenity Prayer
(Children's version)

(We have included the children's version of *The Serenity Prayer*.
It is very powerful and you may want to learn it by heart and say it regularly).

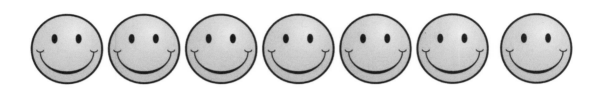

God,

Please make me calm,

So I can accept things,

I cannot change,

Make me brave,

So I can change things I can,

And make me smart enough,

To know the difference.

Amen

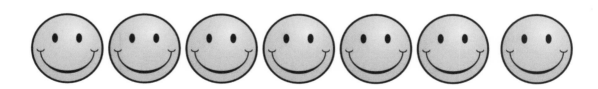

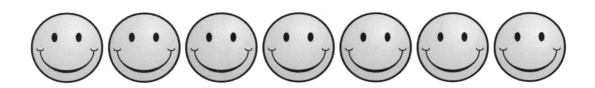

Suggested Book List

- *Bullies Are A Pain in the Brain,* by Trevor Romain and Elizabeth Verdick (age 9-12)

- *Cool Cats, Calm Kids: Relaxation and Stress Management for Young People*, by Mary L. Williams, illustrated by Dianne O'Quinn Burke (age 7 –12)

- *Don't Rant and Rave on Wednesdays: The Children's Anger-Control Book*, by Adolph Moser, illustrated by David Melton (age 9-12)

- *Don't Feed the Monsters on Tuesdays: The Children's Self-Esteem Book*, by Adolph Moser (age 9-12)

- *Don't Pop Your Cork on Mondays: The Children's Anti-Stress Book*, by Adolph Moser, illustrated by Dave Pilkey (age 9-12)

- *Let's Talk About – Feeling Angry,* by Joy Wilt Berry, illustrated by Maggie Smith (age 4-8)

- *Let's Talk About – Feeling Sad,* by Joy Wilt Berry (age 4-8)

- *Let's Talk About – Needing Attention,* by Joy Wilt Berry (age 4-8)

- *Let's Talk About – Saying No,* by Joy Wilt Berry (age 4-8)

- *Psychology for Kids: 40 Fun Tests That Help You Learn About Yourself,* by Jonni Kinder and Julie S. Buck (age 9-12)

- *Stick Up For Yourself: Every Kid's Guide to Personal Power and Positive Self-Esteem,* by Gershen Kaufman and Lev Raphael (age 9-12)

- *What Do You Think: A Kid's Guide to Dealing with Daily   Dilemmas,* by Linda Schwartz and Beverly Armstrong (age 9-12)

- The King County Sexual Assault Resource Center in Washington State offers an excellent brochure entitled, *He Told Me Not To Tell, A parents' guide to talking to children about sexual assault'.* Call (425) 226-5026 for a free copy.

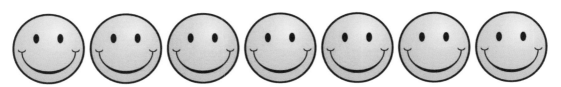

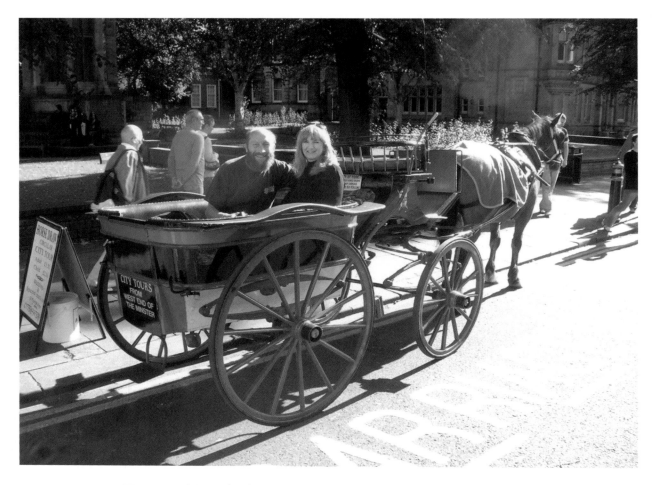

Tom and Marjorie McKinnon in York, England (2006)

The children's version of REPAIR was written by Marjorie McKinnon and illustrated by her husband, Tom McKinnon. They live in northern Arizona along with their Golden Retriever, Guinevere. They have a large family – a small village – living in the Los Angeles area. Marjorie has written twelve manuscripts and five volumes of poetry. The illustration in REPAIR is Tom's first manuscript.

Learn more at her website **www.TheLampLighters.org**

This little exercise book for children who have suffered at the hands and whims of a pedophile or child abuser, has the powerful potential to undo much of the damage done, especially for a child who has no one to turn to for help! The simple exercises are geared towards **empowering** an abused child and **encouraging** that child to thrive before he or she has forever wilted and/or died from the ill-effects of some behavior such as smoking, alcohol, drugs, promiscuity, suicide, eating disorders, cutting or any other self-destructive and self-loathing actions commonly associated with survivors of child abuse.

This book should be left laying around in offices, schools, libraries, arenas and anywhere else children tend to visit – free to be picked up by a child who could benefit. REPAIR should be sponsored and paid for by caring adults or companies and provided for all children to access unconditionally. Even the child who is able to tell needs a program to help them to work their way through their emotional trauma. This book helps the child to re-think and undo the pain and damage caused by bad people!

REMEMBER: Only a tiny fraction of children who are abused ever tell a care-giver, let alone report the crime to authorities because an adult has successfully convinced the child to never tell. Therefore, they are left struggling to help themselves on their own – without resources of any kind.

People who are caring and able should help children to help themselves. If we fail to help, the child falls through the cracks and lives unhappy, unfulfilled and tormented lives. By purchasing copies of this book for access to children in your area, you are providing the child with a life-preserver that could rescue him or her from a wasted life without self-respect or hope! Be a secret hero to a child who is potentially hiding a shameful secret and carrying the heavy burden of guilt that was never theirs.

The harsh reality and truth is;
if you do nothing to stop child abuse,
you are helping children to be abused!

Index

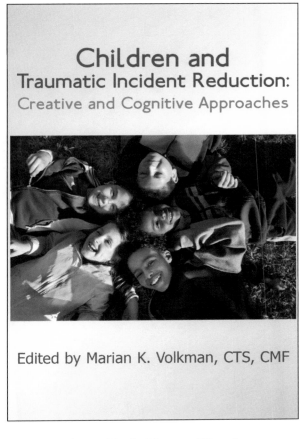

Children and
Traumatic Incident Reduction:
Creative and Cognitive Approaches

Edited by Marian K. Volkman, CTS, CMF

Sam Feels Better Now!
An Interactive Story

Sam saw something awful and scary! Ms. Carol, a special therapist will show Sam how to feel better. Children can help Sam feel better too by using drawings, play, and story telling activities. They will be able to identify and manage their own feelings and difficulties in their lives following a traumatic event.

"This beautiful little picture book is the ideal guide for a series of therapy sessions that will focus the child's attention on positives and help to deal with the traumatic memories."

—Bob Rich, PhD.

"Sam Feels Better Now provides the child and therapist a safe metaphor for exploring trauma issues. The story teaches children that coming to therapy can be a good thing."

—JoAnna White, Ed.D., Chair, Department of Counseling and Psychological Services, Georgia State University

ISBN 978-1-932690-60-6   List $24.95

More information at www.JillOsborne.com

What if we could resolve childhood trauma early, rather than late?

We are understanding more and more about how early traumatic experiences affect long-term mental and physical health:
• Physical impacts are stored in muscles and posture
• Threats of harm are stored as tension
• Overwhelming emotion is held inside
• Negative emotional patterns become habit
• Coping and defense mechanism become inflexible

What if we could resolve childhood trauma before years go by and these effects solidify in body and mind?

In a perfect world, we'd like to be able to shield children from hurt and harm. In the real world, children, even relatively fortunate ones, may experience accidents, injury, illness, and loss of loved ones. Children unfortunate enough to live in unsafe environments live through abuse, neglect, and threats to their well-being and even their life.

Children And Traumatic Incident Reduction
ISBN 978-1-932690-30-9   List $19.95

More information at www.TIRbook.com

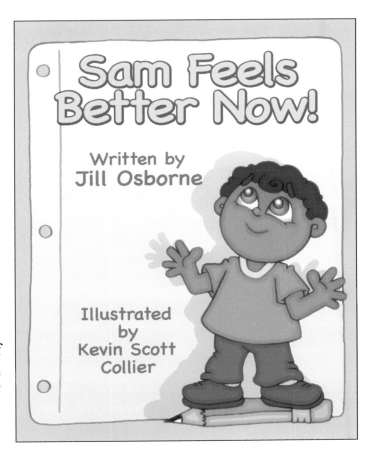

Sam Feels Better Now!

Written by Jill Osborne

Illustrated by Kevin Scott Collier

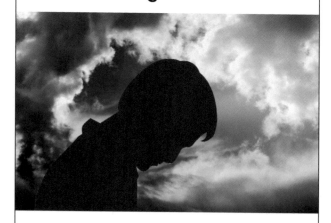

3172077818391

31172077818391

NOV 2 1 2009

LaVergne, TN USA
17 August 2009
154974LV00005B

* 9 7 8 1 9 3 2 6 9 0 5 7